Copyright 2023

Table of Contents

Bronchitis is an inflammation of the lining of your bronchial tubes, which carry air to and from your lungs. People who have bronchitis often cough up thickened mucus, which can be discolored. Bronchitis may be either acute or chronic.

Often developing from a cold or other respiratory infection, acute bronchitis is very common. Chronic bronchitis, a more serious condition, is a constant irritation or inflammation of the lining of the bronchial tubes, often due to smoking.

Acute bronchitis, also called a chest cold, usually improves within a week to 10 days without lasting effects, although the cough may linger for weeks.

However, if you have repeated bouts of bronchitis, you may have chronic bronchitis, which requires medical attention. Chronic bronchitis is one of the conditions included in chronic obstructive pulmonary disease (COPD).

BRONCHITIS DIET RECIPES

BREAKFAST
1. Vegan Instant Pot Chili

Prep Time: 20 Minutes

Cook Time: 30 Minutes

Servings: 6

Ingredient

- 1 (28-oz/800 ml) can of whole tomatoes
- 3 tbsp (45 ml) vegan butter or olive oil
- 1 cup (130 grams) chopped yellow onion (approx. 1 onion)
- 3 cloves garlic, minced
- ½ tbsp (15 ml) all-purpose flour
- 1½ - 2 tablespoon homemade chili powder blend (or substitute store bought)
- 1 tsp (5 ml) paprika
- 1 tsp (5 ml) ground cumin
- 1 tsp (5 ml) dried oregano
- ½ tsp (2.5 ml) ground coriander
- ½ tsp (2.5 ml) garlic powder
- ½ tsp (2.5 ml) onion powder
- ¼ tsp (1.25) cayenne
- ⅛ tsp ground cloves
- 2 cups (500 ml) vegetable broth
- 1 (10-oz/285 ml) can sliced mushrooms, drained and rinsed (approx. 1 cup)
- ½ cup (80 grams) chopped celery (approx. 1 rib)

- ½ cup (75 grams) chopped carrot (approx. 1 carrot)
- ⅔ Cup (100 grams) chopped green bell pepper (approx. ½ pepper)
- 1 tbsp. (15 ml) soy sauce
- ½ tbsp. (7.5 ml) dark brown sugar
- 1 tbsp. (8 grams) of chopped dark chocolate
- 1 (19-oz/540 ml) can cooked red kidney beans, drained and rinsed (approx. 2 cups)
- 1 (19-oz/540 ml) can cooked black beans, drained and rinsed (approx. 1 cup)
- 1 cup (130 grams) or more of vegan ground "beef"
- (I recommend Gardein Beefless Ground)
- Salt, to taste
- Black pepper, to taste

Instructions

1. Drain half of the liquid from the canned tomatoes. Pour half of the tomatoes into a blender and blend smooth. Add the remaining tomatoes and blend briefly, just long enough to chop the tomatoes without blending them smooth.
2. Turn your Instant Pot to the "Sauté" setting on "Normal". Once hot, add the vegan butter. When the butter begins to sizzle, add the onion, garlic, flour, and spices. Cook for 2 minutes.
3. Note: The chili powder blend aroma is strong at this stage but will mellow significantly throughout the cooking process.
4. Stir in the blended tomatoes, vegetable broth, mushrooms, celery, carrot, green pepper, soy sauce, brown sugar, and dark chocolate. Close the Instant Pot

lid securely, (with valve is set to "Sealing") and switch to "Manual" mode (the pressure cooking mode) and set time for 6 minutes.

5. Once the cook time has completed, carefully release the pressure manually (be sure to keep the stream of steam away from your face and hands.) Once it's safe to do so, open the lid.

6. Turn the Instant Pot back to the "Sauté" setting on "Normal". Add the kidney beans, black beans, and vegan ground "beef". Simmer, stirring regularly, until the desired consistency is reached.

7. Taste and adjust the seasoning.

Prep Time: 15 Minutes

Cook Time: 30 Minutes

Servings: 2

Ingredient

Shōyu Ramen Broth:

- 1 tsp sesame oil
- 1 tsp canola oil
- ½ onion
- 4 cloves garlic
- 2 cup mushrooms, slice thick
- 1 ½ tbsp soy sauce
- 1 tsp sriracha
- Pinch dried ginger
- 2 cups vegetable broth

Easy Vegan Ramen:

- 1 package vegan ramen noodles
- ½ package extra-firm tofu, cut into ¼" thick squares
- ½ cup sliced Little Potatoes (Baby Boomers)
- ½ cup sliced mushrooms
- ½ cup baby spinach, julienned
- 1 carrot, in peelings
- 2 green onions, thin sliced
- ½ cup bean sprouts

Instructions

1. Pan-fry extra-firm tofu in sesame or canola oil until crispy on both sides. Set aside.
2. RAMEN BROTH
3. In a medium saucepan, heat sesame + canola oil over medium heat. Add sliced onion and garlic. Cook, stirring frequently, for 1-2 minutes. Add mushrooms and continue cooking until mushrooms are tender. Add ginger, soy sauce, and sriracha, cook, stirring frequently for 1 minute. Slowly add 2 cups vegetable broth. Simmer for 10 minutes, while you prep the ramen toppings.
4. Strain the broth and measure. Add water to correct volume to 600 ml, taste, and adjust with water to suit your preference. Bring broth back to a boil and add sliced potatoes. Simmer for 3 minutes. Add noodles (cooking according to package directions) at the appropriate time to ensure potatoes and noodles are cooked at the same time.
5. RAMEN
6. Divide noodles and broth between 2 bowls. Top with crispy tofu, carrot ribbons, bean sprouts, thin-sliced mushrooms, spinach, and green onion. Serve with sesame seeds, soy sauce, and sriracha.

Prep Time: 20 Minutes

Cook Time: 25 Minutes

Servings: 6

Ingredient

- 1-2 tablespoon (15-30 ml) olive oil, divided
- 1 350g block extra-firm tofu, pressed and cut into cubes
- 2 tbsp (30 ml) soy sauce
- 2 cloves garlic, minced
- ½ cup sliced carrot (approximately 1 carrot)
- ½ cup sliced celery (approximately 1 rib)
- 1 cup (40 grams) kale, stems removed, finely chopped
- 1 cup sliced cremini mushrooms (approximately 5 mushrooms)
- ½ tsp (2.5 ml) ground ginger
- 6 cups (1500 ml) vegetable broth
- ½ cup (50 grams) frozen peas
- 2 cups (170 grams) uncooked pasta (fusilli, farfalle, etc.)

Instructions

1. Cook pasta according to package instructions. Drain and set aside.
2. In a medium-sized bowl, pour soy sauce over cubed tofu. Mix gently until the tofu absorbs the soy sauce.

3. Heat ½ of the olive oil in saucepan over medium-high heat, add tofu and sauté until evenly browned on all (or most) sides.
4. Move the tofu to one side of the pan. Add remaining olive oil and add minced garlic. Cook for 1 minute, do not brown. Add carrot, celery, kale, mushrooms, and ground ginger. Stir and cook for 3 minutes.
5. Add the vegetable broth and simmer for 5 minutes.
6. Add frozen peas and simmer for another 3-5 minutes, or until the vegetables are just tender.
7. Taste and adjust seasoning.
8. Keep pasta and soup separate until ready to serve. Divide cooked pasta into bowls and top with hot soup.

Prep Time: 5 Minutes

Cook Time: 15 Minutes

Servings: 4

Ingredient

- 1 ½ cups (225 g) elbow macaroni
- ¾ cups (175 ml) unsweetened non-dairy milk
- ⅔ cup (60 g) vegan cheese shreds (I used Follow Your Heart/Earth Island Mozzarella)
- 2 tbsp (30 ml) vegan butter or margarine
- 2 tbsp (8 g) nutritional yeast flakes
- 2-3 teaspoon (10-15 ml) white vinegar
- 1 tsp (5 ml) garlic powder
- 1 tsp (5 ml) onion powder
- 1-2 teaspoon (5-10 ml) sugar
- ½ tsp (2.5 ml) salt, add more to taste
- Black pepper, to taste

Instructions

1. In a small bowl, measure out the cheese, butter, nutritional yeast, vinegar, garlic and onion powder, sugar, and salt.
2. Bring a large pot of heavily salted water to boil. Add macaroni noodles. Cook pasta al dent, according to package instructions. Drain the pasta but DO NOT rinse it. The leftover starch from cooking the pasta thickens the cheese sauce.

3. In the pot you used to boil the pasta, turn heat to medium. Add the cooked macaroni, and stir in unsweetened almond milk, and measured ingredients from step 1. The mac and cheese will look a little soupy at this stage.
4. Continue cooking, stirring constantly, until vegan cheese is melted, and the sauce is smooth and thickened to your liking. Taste and adjust seasoning.

Prep Time: 15 Minutes

Cook Time: 35 Minutes

Servings: 7

Ingredient

- 3 tbsp/45ml olive oil
- 1 block (350g) extra-firm tofu, cubed
- 2 tbsp (30ml) soy sauce
- ½ cup/125ml (100g) chopped yellow onion (1 onion)
- 1 ½ cups/375ml (200g) chopped carrots (4 carrots)
- 1 ½ cups (185g) chopped celery (3 ribs celery)
- 2 cloves garlic, minced
- 1 - 1.5lb bag (680g) of The Little Potato Company's Fingerling potatoes
- ½ cup/125ml (75g) unbleached flour
- 6 cups/1500ml vegetable broth
- 1 cup/250ml water
- 3 tbsp/45ml tomato paste
- 1 pinch dried thyme
- 1 cup/250ml (140g) frozen peas

Instructions

1. With the lid off, turn Instant Pot on to "Sauté" and choose the "Normal" heat level. Add the olive oil. Once the Instant Pot is preheated, add the cubed tofu. Cook, stirring occasionally, until the tofu is crisp and golden brown on all sides, about 10 minutes.

2. Add the soy sauce and stir, cooking until the liquid is absorbed.
3. Add the onion, carrot, celery, and garlic. Stir and cook for 2 minutes.
4. Add the flour and mix well. Cook for 2 minutes, stirring often.
5. Add the Fingerling potatoes, vegetable broth, water, tomato paste, and thyme. Stir well.
6. Securely close the lid on your Instant Pot and turn it on to "Manual" or "Pressure Cook". Set timer for 15 minutes.
7. Once finished, release the pressure (following Instant Pot instructions) and open the lid when safe to do so.
8. Add the frozen peas and stir. With the lid off, use the "Sauté" functions set to a heat level of "More" or "High" and reduce the stew to your preferred thickness, about 5 minutes.
9. Taste and adjust seasoning.

Prep Time: 40 Minutes

Cook Time: 1hr 40 Minutes

Servings: 5

Ingredient

Pastry Crust:

- 1 ⅓ cups (160 grams) all purpose flour
- Pinch salt
- ½ cup (115 grams) chilled vegetable shortening or vegan butter
- 2-3 tablespoon (30 - 45 ml) ice water

Vegan Pot Pie Filling:

- ½ (350g/14-oz block) firm tofu, pressed and cubed
- 1 tbsp (15 ml) soy sauce
- 3 tbsp (45 ml) vegan butter or vegetable oil, divided (plus extra for brushing)
- ⅔ cup (90 grams) chopped carrot (approx. 1 carrot)
- ⅓ cup (50 grams) chopped celery (approx. 1 rib)
- ½ cup (70 grams) chopped onion (approx. ½ onion)
- 1 clove garlic, minced
- ¼ cup (35 grams) all-purpose flour
- 1 cup (250 ml) vegetable broth
- 1 ¼ cup (310 ml) original non-dairy milk
- ¾ cup (125 grams) chopped Creamer potatoes (any variety by The Little Potato Company)
- ½ tsp (2.5 ml) garlic powder
- ½ tsp (2.5 ml) onion powder

- ¼ tsp (1.25 ml) dried thyme
- ¼ cup (50 grams) frozen peas
- ½ tsp (2.5 ml) white wine vinegar
- Salt and pepper, to taste

Instructions

Pastry Crust:

1. Mix flour and salt in a medium mixing bowl. Cut the chilled shortening into the flour using a pastry blender, until the fat is uniformly combined and the mixture begins to stick together.
2. Add 2-3 tablespoon of ice water and stir just enough for the mixture to form a dough. Wrap the dough tightly in plastic wrap and refrigerate while you prepare the filling.
3. After chilling, cut the dough into 4 or 6 equal pieces. Form each piece into a round disk. On a floured surface, roll each piece of dough out into a roughly circular shape, slightly larger than your ramekins. Cut off any excess to make a round.

Vegan Pot Pie Filling and Assembly:

1. Preheat oven to 400°F (200°C).
2. Mix cubed tofu and soy sauce together. In a large skillet or dutch oven, heat 1 tablespoon butter over medium heat. Add cubed tofu/soy sauce and cook, stirring and turning often until browned on all sides. Remove tofu from pan and set aside.
3. In the same pan, heat 2 tablespoon of vegan butter over medium heat. Once it begins to sizzle, add the carrot, celery, onion, and garlic. Cook for 2 minutes.

4. Stir in the flour and cook, stirring constantly, for 1 minute.
5. Gradually add vegetable broth and non-dairy milk, stirring constantly to prevent lumps.
6. Add the Little potatoes, tofu, garlic powder, onion powder, and thyme. Simmer for 10 minutes. Begin rolling out the pie dough while the filling simmers.
7. Stir in the frozen peas and white wine vinegar. Taste and adjust seasoning with salt and pepper.
8. Divide filling into 6 (½ cup / 125 ml capacity) ramekins. Top with pie crust, folding the crust over the edges of the ramekin. Brush with melted vegan butter or non-dairy milk. Poke a few holes in the crust to allow steam to escape.

Prep Time: 30 Minutes

Cook Time: 10 Minutes

Servings: 2

Ingredient

Lemon Poppy Seed Scones:

- 1 ¾ cups unbleached all-purpose flour
- 1 ½ tbsp granulated sugar
- ½ tbsp baking powder
- ½ tsp baking soda
- ½ tsp salt
- 1 tbsp poppy seeds
- Zest of 1 lemon (finely chopped)
- ¼ cup coconut oil (chilled)
- ¾ cup + 1 tbsp Silk Unsweetened Organic Soymilk

Lemon Glaze:

- 1 tbsp coconut oil (melted)
- 2 tbsp Silk Unsweetened Organic Soymilk (warm)
- 10 ml lemon juice
- ¾ cup icing sugar
- 1 tbsp lemon zest

Instructions

Lemon Poppy Seed Scones:

1. Preheat oven to 400F.

2. Combine all dry ingredients, including poppy seeds and lemon zest.

3. Add the chilled coconut oil to the dry ingredients. Use your hands to cut the coconut oil into the dry ingredients. Continue working the coconut oil into the dry ingredients until the mixture resembles fine crumbs. (I find it helpful to chill my hands by rinsing them under very cold water for a minute or so. This will help you break up the coconut oil without melting it.)

4. Add the soy milk and use a fork to stir the ingredients. Do NOT over mix. As soon as the mixture is just combined, turn it onto a floured kitchen counter. Knead about 8-12 times before rolling out on a well-floured counter. The dough should be about 1" thick. Cut into rustic triangles (about the size of a deck of cards.)

5. Transfer to a parchment paper lined baking sheet (leaving at least ½" between scones) and bake for 10 minutes. They should be golden brown.

6. Cool before glazing.

Glaze:

1. Combine the warm soy milk, coconut oil, lemon juice, icing sugar, and lemon zest. Whisk until combined. Add more soy milk for a thinner glaze (good for dunking the entire scone), add more icing sugar for a thicker glaze (great for drizzling). Once the scones are cooled, drizzle or dunk in glaze. Enjoy!

Prep Time: 25 Minutes

Cook Time: 15 Minutes

Servings: 25

Ingredient

- 1 cup (240 grams) vegan butter (I used Earth Balance)
- ½ cup (120 grams) sugar
- 1 teaspoon (5 ml) vanilla extract
- ¼ teaspoon (1.25 ml) salt
- 3 tablespoons (45 ml) Aquafina
- 2 ½ cups (300 grams) all-purpose flour see notes

Instructions

2. Preheat oven to 350°F (180°C).
3. In a large bowl or stand mixer, cream together vegan butter and sugar until light and fluffy.
4. Add vanilla, salt, and Aquafina to the creamed butter mixture and beat for 5 minutes.
5. Mixing by hand, gradually add the flour. Mix until the dough is just blended. Avoid over mixing. The dough should be just firm but not stiff.
6. Fill a large piping bag fitted with a large star tip (or a cookie press), with the cookie dough. Pipe or press the cookies onto a cool cookie sheet, leaving a little space for the cookies to spread.
7. If desired, sprinkle cookies with colored sanding sugar or top with a glacé cherry.

8. Bake until the cookies are just golden-brown around the edges, about 10-13 minutes.
9. Transfer cookies to a cooling rack and allow to cool completely.
10. For best texture, store vegan butter cookies lightly wrapped for 1 day before transferring to an airtight container. Freezer-friendly.

Prep Time: 2hr 30 Minutes

Cook Time: 00 Minutes

Servings: 1

Ingredient

- 2 cups (240 grams) all-purpose flour
- ¼ tsp (1.25 ml) salt
- ¾ cup (170 grams) vegan butter (Earth Balance Buttery Spread)
- 4-8 tablespoon (60-120 ml) ice water

Instructions

1. Before you get started, chill all ingredients and tools.
2. Mix the flour and salt in a medium mixing bowl.
3. Cut the chilled vegan butter into the flour using a pastry blender or fork until the fat is in small pieces.
4. Slowly add ice water, 1 tablespoon at a time, while gently mixing with a fork. Keep adding the water and stirring until the vegan pie dough starts to clump together on its own. The dough should look crumbly, but hold together. The dough shouldn't be wet or sticky.
5. On your countertop, lay out a piece of plastic wrap (I use 2, laid out in a cross shape.) Dump the crumbly vegan pie dough in the center of the plastic wrap. Very tightly wrap the dough into a flat disk so that the dough doesn't appear crumbly at all. Refrigerate for 2 hours before rolling out.

6. After chilling the dough, unwrap it and place it on a liberally floured surface. Start rolling from the center of the dough, out to the edges. Roll out the pie dough in different directions to achieve a roughly circular shape.

7. Roll out the dough until the dough is at least 2 inches larger than your pie plate. Gently lift the pie dough from your work surface using your metal spatula, and transfer it to your pie plate.

8. Making sure the dough lays flush with your pie plate, all the way into the corners. Leave 1 inch (2.5 cm) of excess for folding and fluting the edges, and cut away the rest.

9. Use your fingers to gently mend any cracks by lightly pinching and massaging them to smooth them out.

10. Slowly and gently fold the excess dough under itself to make a smooth, clean edge, folded on the lip of your pie plate.

11. Use the thumb and index finger of your dominant hand and the thumb of your non-dominant hand to pinch/flute the edge of your pie crust. Use a fork to pierce holes in the bottom of the crust.

12. Chill or freeze your pie crust until ready to use.

Prep Time: 25 Minutes

Cook Time: 25 Minutes

Servings: 15

Ingredient

Focaccia:

- 1½ cups (375 ml) warm water
- 1 tbsp (15 ml) sugar
- 1 tbsp (15 ml) active dry yeast
- 1 tsp (5 ml) salt
- 4½ cups (540 grams) all-purpose flour
- Olive oil, as needed

Toppings:

- Jalapeño & Cheese Option (1 full sheet pan)
- 1 cup (140 grams) pickled (tamed) jalapeños
- ½ cup (45 grams) vegan cheese shreds (I used Daiya)
- 4 cloves garlic, thinly sliced
- Optional: vegan Parmesan, to taste
- Sea salt, to taste
- Tomato & Herb Option (1 full sheet pan)
- 1 cup (160 grams) halved grape or cherry tomatoes
- 4 cloves garlic, thinly sliced
- Fresh or dried Italian herbs (oregano, thyme, rosemary, basil, etc.), to taste
- Sea salt, to taste

Instructions

1. In a large bowl or stand mixer, combine warm water, sugar, yeast, salt, and ¾ of the all-purpose flour. Mix to combine. Knead (by hand or in a stand mixer with a dough hook) until the dough is smooth and elastic (about 10 minutes), add remaining flour as needed to keep the dough from sticking.
2. Coat the dough ball with olive oil and place it in a large bowl covered with a damp kitchen towel. Leave to rise until doubled in size (about 1 hour).
3. Line a large baking sheet with parchment paper. Drizzle the parchment paper with olive oil.
4. After the dough doubles in size, punch it down. Flatten and stretch the dough to fit your sheet pan. Cover lightly with a sheet of plastic wrap and let rise until doubled in size (about 40 minutes).
5. While the dough rises, preheat your oven to 450°F (230°C) and prepare toppings.
6. After the dough has risen, add your choice of toppings. Use your fingers to thoroughly dimple the dough, pressing the toppings into the bread. Drizzle with olive oil and season with sea salt.
7. Bake focaccia until golden brown, about 25-30 minutes.

11. Fudgy Vegan Brownies

Prep Time: 25 Minutes

Cook Time: 25 Minutes

Servings: 15

Ingredient

Brownies:

- ⅔ Cup coconut oil
- 180g chopped vegan dark chocolate
- ½ cup Aquafina (the juice from a can of "no salt added" chickpeas)
- ¾ cup + 2 tbsp golden brown sugar
- 1 ¾ cup + 2 tbsp unbleached all-purpose flour
- ¼ cup cocoa
- ¾ tsp salt
- ½ tsp baking soda
- 2 tbsp espresso or strong black coffee
- ½ cup vegan chocolate chips
- ½ cup chopped walnuts
- Magic Shell
- 1 tbsp coconut oil
- 50g dark chocolate

Instructions

1. Preheat oven to 325F. Line an 8"x 8"pan with parchment paper.

2. In a stand mixer, beat the Aquafina and brown sugar on high until it becomes thick, shiny, and voluminous.
3. In a double boiler over medium heat, combine the chocolate and coconut oil. Stir until completely melted and set aside to cool. (For quicker cooling, place the bowl in an ice bath and stir constantly until the chocolate is no longer warm.)
4. Sift together the flour, cocoa, sea salt and baking soda.
5. Gently mix the cooled, melted chocolate into whipped Aquafina/sugar mixture, followed by the espresso, and then the dry ingredients. Add the walnuts and chocolate chips. Stir slowly until the batter is thick and well combined.
6. Pour batter into prepared pan and bake for 22 minutes, or until a toothpick inserted into the center comes out clean. Optional: Top with extra chopped walnuts.
7. Magic Shell: Melt coconut oil and dark chocolate in a double boiler or microwave.

Prep Time: 15 Minutes

Cook Time: 1hr 10 Minutes

Servings: 1

Ingredient

- ½ cup (125 ml) non-dairy milk
- 2 tbsp (15 grams) ground flax seed
- 1 cup packed (155 grams) grated zucchini (approximately 1 medium zucchini)
- 1 cup (225 grams) sugar
- ⅓ cup (80 ml) canola oil
- 1 tsp (5 ml) vanilla extract
- 1 ½ cups (180 grams) all-purpose flour
- ⅓ cup (30 grams) natural cocoa powder (do not substitute with Dutch processed/alkalized cocoa)
- ¾ tsp (3.75 ml) baking soda
- ½ tsp (2.5 ml) salt
- Dark chocolate chunks or chocolate chips, to taste (Optional)

Instructions

1. Preheat the oven to 350°F (177°C). Line a loaf pan with parchment paper.
2. In a medium-sized bowl, combine non-dairy milk and flax. Set aside for 5 minutes.
3. In a large bowl, sift together the flour, natural cocoa powder, baking soda, and salt. Mix and set aside.

4. Once the milk and flax seed mixture has thickened slightly, add the grated zucchini, sugar, canola oil, and vanilla to the bowl.

5. Once the oven is preheated, stir the wet ingredients into the dry ingredients. Immediately transfer the batter into the parchment lined loaf pan. If desired, top with chocolate chunks. Immediately put the loaf in the oven and bake for 70 minutes (or until the loaf is cracked and a toothpick inserted in the center comes out clean.)

6. Transfer zucchini loaf to a cooling rack. Wait until cool to slice the loaf. Store in an air-tight container.

Prep Time: 20 Minutes

Cook Time: 25 Minutes

Servings: 7

Ingredient

- Approximately 3 lemons, zester and juiced, divided
- Powdered sugar, for dusting

Shortbread Crust

- 1 cup (230 grams) vegan butter
- ½ cup (60 grams) powdered sugar
- 1 tbsp lemon zest
- ⅛ tsp salt
- 2 cups (240 grams) all-purpose flour

Lemon Layer

- ½ cup (125 ml) fresh lemon juice
- ¼ cup (35 grams) cornstarch
- ¾ cup (185 ml) canned coconut cream or full fat coconut milk*
- 1 cup (215 grams) sugar
- ½ cup (115 grams) vegan butter (like Earth Balance or Melt)
- 3 tbsp lemon zest
- ⅛ tsp salt
- Pinch turmeric

Instructions

Shortbread Crust:

1. Preheat oven to 350°F (180°C).
2. Line a 9x13 baking dish with parchment paper.
3. Cream together vegan butter, powdered sugar, lemon zest, and salt. Gradually mix in the flour to create a soft dough. Do not over mix.
4. Press the dough into the bottom of your baking dish.
5. Bake the crust for 20-25 minutes or until golden. Prepare the filling as the crust bakes.

Lemon Layer:

1. In a medium saucepan, whisk together the lemon juice and cornstarch to make a slurry. Make sure there are no lumps. Whisk in the coconut milk and add the sugar, vegan butter, lemon zest, and salt.
2. Turn heat to medium and stir until the sugar and butter melts. Whisk in the turmeric, adding a small pinch at a time, until you achieve a light yellow color.
3. Cook the filling, whisking constantly. Make sure to scrape the bottom and sides of the pot to prevent lumps. Cook the filling until its thick and slightly translucent (about 15 minute's total). Once the filling begins to bubble, test it for doneness by stirring it and quickly removing your whisk - once the lines from your whisk stay visible for 7-10 seconds after pulling it out, the filling is thick enough.
4. Pour the lemon filling over the shortbread crust. Set bars aside to cool slightly before chilling, uncovered. Once chilled, slice lemon bars. Dust with powdered sugar just prior to serving.

Prep Time: 15 Minutes

Cook Time: 60 Minutes

Servings: 1

Ingredient

- 1 ½ cups (365 g) mashed overripe banana (approx. 3 large bananas)
- ¾ cup (175 ml) (150 g) granulated sugar
- ⅓ cup (80 ml) canola oil
- 3 tbsp (45 ml) unsweetened non-dairy milk (I used oat)
- 2 tbsp (30 ml) (10 g) ground flax seed
- 2 tsp (10 ml) white vinegar
- 1 tsp (5 ml) vanilla
- 1 ¾ cup (210 g) all-purpose flour see recipe notes
- 1 tsp (5 ml) baking powder
- 1 tsp (5 ml) baking soda
- ½ tsp (2.5 ml) ground cinnamon
- ½ tsp (2.5 ml) salt
- ½ cup (90 g) mini dairy-free chocolate chips (optional)
- ½-1 cup chopped walnuts or pecans (optional)

Instructions

1. Preheat oven to 350°F (177°C) and line a loaf pan with parchment paper. After that, there's no need to wait for your oven to preheat fully before moving on to steps 2 and 3.

2. Use a fork to mash the over ripe bananas. Don't worry about thoroughly mashing them, its okay if there are still chunks of banana.

3. In a large bowl, whisk together mashed banana, sugar, canola oil, non-dairy milk, ground flax seeds, vinegar, and vanilla. Then, let the mixture sit until the oven is preheated.

4. In the same bowl, use a whisk to mix in the flour, baking powder, baking soda, cinnamon, and salt.

5. Optional: Stir in chocolate chips.

6. Pour the batter into the loaf pan lined with parchment paper.

7. Bake for 50-60 minutes or until the loaf is a deep golden-brown color and a toothpick inserted into the center comes out clean.

8. Remove from oven and let cool in the pan for 5 minutes. After that remove the vegan banana bread from the pan and cool on a cooling rack. When the loaf is just barely warm, seal it up in a container, food storage bag, or plastic wrap for a couple of hours or until the crust becomes soft and moist.

9. Wait until completely cool before slicing and serving with vegan butter.

10. Store in a sealed container or food storage bag for 5 days. Do not refrigerate.

Prep Time: 20 Minutes

Cook Time: 22 Minutes

Servings: 12

Ingredient

Vegan Chocolate Cupcakes:

- 1 cup / 250ml / (135g) unbleached all-purpose flour
- 1 ¼ cups / 310ml / (266g) granulated sugar
- ½ cup / 125ml / (40g) cocoa powder
- ¾ tsp / 3.75ml baking powder
- ¼ tsp / 1.25ml baking soda

Pinch salt:

- 1 cup / 250ml soy milk (any kind: unsweetened, original, vanilla, etc.)
- ⅓ cup / 80ml canola oil
- 1 tsp / 5ml vanilla extract
- ½ tsp / 2.5ml white vinegar

Vegan Buttercream Frosting

- 1 cup / 250ml / (220g) vegan butter, slightly softened at room temperature
- 4-5 cups / 1000ml-1250ml / (560g-700g) icing sugar
- 1 tbsp / 15ml vanilla extract

Instructions

Vegan Chocolate Cupcakes:

1. Preheat oven to 350°F (177°C).
2. Prepare muffin tin with cupcake liners. If not using cupcake liners, grease muffin tin with non-stick spray or canola oil and dust with flour.
3. Combine dry ingredients in a medium-sized bowl.
4. Add wet ingredients to dry ingredients. Whisk for 3 minutes.
5. Equally divide batter into muffin tins.
6. Bake for 22 minutes. Test with a toothpick inserted into the center of cupcake, it should come out clean.
7. After baking, let cupcakes sit for 10 minutes before transferring to a cooling rack.
8. Wait until cupcakes are cool before frosting (approx. 1 hour at room temperature.)
9. VEGAN BUTTERCREAM FROSTING
10. Use a stand mixer or hand mixer to cream butter until soft and fluffy.
11. Add vanilla and mix.
12. Add icing sugar, ½ cup at a time, until the frosting is light and fluffy. Keep in mind that the buttercream frosting will get softer as it warms up.
13. Optional: Add food coloring and mix until you achieve your desired color.
14. Optional: If piping the buttercream frosting onto cupcakes, transfer it to a piping bag.
15. Chill in refrigerator until ready to use.

Prep Time: 10 Minutes

Cook Time: 20 Minutes

Servings: 2

Ingredient

Garlic Roasted Broccoli:

- 2 cups broccoli
- 2 tsp olive or canola oil
- 2 cloves garlic, minced
- Pinch of salt
- Black pepper

Roasted Sriracha & Soy Sauce Chickpeas:

- 1.5 cups (cooked) chickpeas
- 1 tsp olive or canola oil
- 2 tsp sriracha
- 2 tsp soy sauce

Curry Roasted Sweet Potatoes

- 1 small sweet potato
- 1 tsp olive or canola oil
- 1 tsp curry powder
- 1 tsp sriracha
- Pinch salt

Quinoa

- ¾ cup quinoa, rinsed
- 1.5 cups vegetable broth

Chili-Lime Kale

- 2 cups (packed) kale, DE stemmed and chopped
- 1 tsp olive, coconut or canola oil
- Juice of ¼ lime
- ½ tsp chili powder
- Pinch salt
- Pinch pepper
- OPTIONAL
- Lime
- Avocado
- Hummus
- Red pepper flakes
- Guacamole

Instructions

Roasting:

1. Preheat oven to 400F. Line a large baking sheet with parchment paper.
2. Prep your vegetables: chop broccoli into medium sized florets, esteem and chop the kale, scrub and slice the sweet potato into ¼" wide rounds.
3. Massage the broccoli florets with oil, garlic, salt and pepper - make sure to work the ingredients into the tops of the florets. Lay them in a row down the center third of a large baking sheet.
4. Using the same bowl you mixed the broccoli in, combine chickpeas, oil, sriracha and soy sauce. Spread them out in a row next to the broccoli.
5. In the same bowl combine the oil, curry powder, salt, and sriracha. Add the sliced sweet potato and toss to

coat. Lay the rounds on the remaining third of the baking tray.

6. Bake for 10 minutes. Flip the broccoli and sweet potatoes and redistribute the chickpeas to promote even cooking. Bake for another 8-12 minutes.

Quinoa:

1. Rinse and drain the quinoa. Add rinsed quinoa and vegetable broth to a small saucepan and bring to a boil over high heat. Turn the heat down to medium-low, cover and simmer for approx. 15 minutes. Once cooked, fluff with a fork and set aside.

Kale:

2. While the quinoa is simmering and the rest of the ingredients are roasting, preheat a large skillet with 1 teaspoon oil. Add the kale and cook for approx. 5 minutes, or until nearly tender. Add the salt, chili powder, and lime juice. Toss to coat and cook for another 2-3 minutes.

Serving:

3. Assemble the bowls: Scoop ½ to 1 cup of quinoa into each bowl, top with ½ of the broccoli, ½ the chickpeas, ½ kale, and ½ sweet potatoes. Feel free to keep everything separated in the bowl or mix it all together.

Prep Time: 20 Minutes

Cook Time: 25 Minutes

Servings: 6

Ingredient

- 1-2 tablespoon (15-30 ml) olive oil, divided
- 1 350g block extra-firm tofu, pressed and cut into cubes
- 2 tbsp (30 ml) soy sauce
- 2 cloves garlic, minced
- ½ cup sliced carrot (approximately 1 carrot)
- ½ cup sliced celery (approximately 1 rib)
- 1 cup (40 grams) kale, stems removed, finely chopped
- 1 cup sliced cremini mushrooms (approximately 5 mushrooms)
- ½ tsp (2.5 ml) ground ginger
- 6 cups (1500 ml) vegetable broth
- ½ cup (50 grams) frozen peas
- 2 cups (170 grams) uncooked pasta (fusilli, farfalle, etc.)

Instructions

4. Cook pasta according to package instructions. Drain and set aside.
5. In a medium-sized bowl, pour soy sauce over cubed tofu. Mix gently until the tofu absorbs the soy sauce.

6. Heat ½ of the olive oil in saucepan over medium-high heat, add tofu and sauté until evenly browned on all (or most) sides.
7. Move the tofu to one side of the pan. Add remaining olive oil and add minced garlic. Cook for 1 minute, do not brown. Add carrot, celery, kale, mushrooms, and ground ginger. Stir and cook for 3 minutes.
8. Add the vegetable broth and simmer for 5 minutes.
9. Add frozen peas and simmer for another 3-5 minutes, or until the vegetables are just tender.
10. Taste and adjust seasoning.
11. Keep pasta and soup separate until ready to serve. Divide cooked pasta into bowls and top with hot soup.

18. Vegan Rice Paper Rolls with Sriracha & Soy Sauce Tofu (Served with A Spicy-Sweet Peanut Sauce!)

Prep Time: 45 Minutes

Cook Time: oo Minutes

Servings: 8

Ingredient

Fresh Vegetable Crunchy Rolls with Sriracha & Soy Sauce Tofu:

- ½ red pepper, julienned
- 1 large carrot, julienned
- ⅓ -½ long English cucumber, julienned
- 3 green onions, thinly sliced on a diagonal
- small handful of baby spinach, gently bunched up and sliced thinly
- ½-1 full recipe of Baked Sriracha & Soy Sauce Tofu (optional: double the marinade), chilled and cut into thin strips
- Sesame seeds
- 6-9 rice papers (I used 22 cm papers)

Peanut Sauce:

- 2 tbsp (30 ml) soy sauce (or Bragg's Liquid Aminos - GF)
- 3 tbsp (45 ml) peanut butter
- 1 tbsp (15 ml) sriracha
- 1 tbsp (15 ml) chili garlic sauce (can substitute with 1 more tablespoon sriracha)
- 1 tbsp (15 ml) sesame oil

- 1 tbsp (15 ml) brown sugar (or maple syrup)
- 1 tbsp (15 ml) sesame seeds
- 2-3 tbsp (30-45ml) water to thin

Instructions

Fresh Vegetable Crunchy Rolls with Sriracha & Soy Sauce Tofu:

1. While the tofu is baking you can begin to prepare all of your ingredients. Finely julienne the red pepper, carrot, and cucumber (you can use a julienne peeler for the carrot and cucumber as well) I aim for slices between 4-5 inches long (but this depends on the size of your rice paper, mine are about 8" (20 cm).) Thinly slice the spinach and green onion.
2. Once the tofu has finished baking, place it in the fridge to chill. In the meantime you can mix up the Spicy-Sweet Peanut Sauce (recipe below.)
3. Cut your chilled tofu into thin strips.
4. Prep your area. Find a nice clean space of counter to work on and fill a large bowl or pie plate with HOT water. Grab your sesame seeds and all of your prepped veggies.

Assembly:

1. Soak a single rice paper in the hot water until it's completely soft and flexible. This could take anywhere from a few seconds to more than 30 seconds depending on the brand/type of rice paper. I have best results soaking them for about 30 seconds.

2. Gently shake the excess water from the rice paper, lay it straight out onto your work space.
3. Let it sit for about 30 seconds to absorb any excess water, the papers won't stick together properly if they're really wet.
4. Sprinkle some sesame seeds in the center of the wrap.
5. Lay the julienned vegetables down in the middle of the wrap. Use approximately ⅕ of each ingredients per wrap (use a little more or a little less deepening on how many wraps you want to make and how big you'd like them to be.) I like to fill mine with a little bit of spinach, lots of cucumber and carrot, a little red pepper, and lots of tofu topped with a sprinkle of green onion.
6. Try to keep the fillings laid neatly, making sure to leave ample room on each side to easily fold the wrap.

Rolling:

1. Lift the side of the rice paper that's closest to you, gently pull it forward (away from you) over the fillings. Hold the wrap firmly while you fold in each end of the wrap. Continue rolling to seal the seam. Refer to the GIF above for a demo.

Spicy-Sweet Peanut Sauce:

2. Combine all ingredients in a bowl and whisk vigorously OR combine all ingredients in food processor and pulse.
3. Store extra sauce in the fridge. I like to keep mine in a glass salad dressing bottle. It may thicken up when refrigerated, I just run my bottle under hot running tap water until it softens back to a liquid.
4. Makes approx. ½ cup of sauce.

Prep Time: 15 Minutes

Cook Time: 35 Minutes

Servings: 8

Ingredient

Creamy Vegan Broccoli Soup:

- ¼ cup (60 ml) vegan butter or olive oil
- 5 cups (360 grams) broccoli, chopped (approx. 2 heads)
- ⅔ cup (100 grams) chopped carrots (approx. 2 carrots)
- ⅔ cup (100 grams) chopped celery (approx. 2 ribs)
- ⅔ cups (100 grams) chopped onion, (approx. 1 onion)
- 2 cloves garlic, minced
- 6 tbsp (65 grams) flour
- 4 cups (1000 ml) vegetable broth
- 2 cups (500 ml) original or unsweetened non-dairy milk (I recommend original cashew)
- ¾ cup (185 ml) full-fat canned coconut milk (or sub with more non-dairy milk)
- ¼ cup (20 grams) nutritional yeast flakes (or sub with vegan cheese shreds)
- 1 tsp (5 ml) white wine vinegar or lemon juice
- ½ tsp (2.5 ml) salt, to taste
- Black pepper, to taste

Browned Broccoli "Croutons"

- 1 cup (70 grams) broccoli florets
- 1 tbsp (15 ml) olive oil

- Salt, to taste

Instructions

Creamy Vegan Broccoli Soup

1. In a medium saucepan, heat vegan butter or olive oil over medium heat. Add the broccoli, carrot, celery, onion, and garlic. Sauté until onion is translucent and just tender, about 5 minutes.
2. Sprinkle vegetables with flour. Cook for 1-2 minutes, stirring often.
3. Gradually add vegetable broth and non-dairy milk, stirring constantly to prevent lumps. Add the coconut milk and nutritional yeast. Simmer soup over medium-low heat for 10-15 minutes, or until the vegetables are tender.
4. Blend the soup to your liking. I recommend puréeing ½ to ⅔ of the soup smooth.
5. If desired, adjust consistency with vegetable broth or non-dairy milk. Stir in white wine vinegar. Taste and adjust seasoning with salt, pepper, vinegar, (and if desired, sugar if using unsweetened non-dairy milk - refer to recipe notes).

Browned Broccoli Croutons:

1. In a separate saucepan or skillet, heat olive oil over medium heat.
2. Add the broccoli florets and sprinkle with salt. Sauté until just nearly tender. Turn the heat up to high and continue to cook, stirring sporadically, until the broccoli has a nice brown/black edge on at least 1 side. Remove from heat and set aside.

Serving:

1. Ladle soup into bowls. Drizzle with a little bit of olive oil, top with browned broccoli florets, vegan cheese shreds (optional),and cracked black pepper. Serve with crackers, bread, sandwich or salad. Enjoy!

Prep Time: 00 Minutes

Cook Time: 00 Minutes

Servings: 4

Ingredient

- 2 cups packed, grated, and drained potato (half of a 1.5 lb bag of The Little Potato Company's Baby Boomers)
- ⅓ cup unbleached all-purpose flour
- 3 tbsp sliced green onion
- 3 tbsp unsweetened nondairy milk
- 1 tbsp cornstarch
- 1 ¼ tsp salt
- ½ tsp baking powder
- black pepper, to taste
- vegetable oil, for frying (canola, olive, or coconut all work well)
- optional: 2 tablespoon fresh, chopped dill
- optional: ¼ cup vegan cheese shreds

Instructions

1. Grate potatoes and squeeze out as much moisture as you can using paper towel.
2. Combine 2 cups grated potato, flour, green onion, almond milk, cornstarch, salt, baking powder, and black pepper (optional: add dill and vegan cheese.) Mix well to develop the gluten in the flour (which helps with binding.)

3. In a frying pan, preheat a generous amount of vegetable oil over medium heat.

4. Spoon ¼-1/3 cup of potato mixture into the pan. Use a spatula or pancake flipper to flatten the patty to about ¼" thick. Fry until golden brown, flip, and fry the other side. Drain excess oil on paper towel if necessary.

5. Serve with your favorite toppings (we used sliced green onion, tzatziki, and black pepper.)

Prep Time: 00 Minutes

Cook Time: 00 Minutes

Servings: 2

Ingredient

Couscous:

- 1 cup whole wheat couscous
- 1 cup vegetable broth
- 1 tsp. soy sauce

Tofu:

- 1 block (350g.) extra-firm tofu, drained and cubed
- 1 ½ tbsp. cornstarch
- ¼ tsp. sea salt
- ¼ tsp. garlic powder

Oil, for frying

Garlicky Cashew Broccoli:

- 1 ½ tbsp. brown sugar
- 1 tbsp. hot water
- 2 tbsp. soy sauce
- ½ tsp. lemon juice
- 2 tbsp. vegan butter (divided)
- 4 cups, (227g.) broccoli florets
- ½ cup, (64g.) chopped or halved raw cashews
- 3 cloves garlic, minced

- To serve: sriracha, sesame seeds, etc.

Instructions

Couscous:

1. Prepare couscous according to package instructions, substituting 1 cup vegetable broth and 1 tsp. soy sauce for every cup of water required.

Tofu:

2. In a medium-sized bowl, combine drained, cubed tofu, cornstarch, salt, and garlic powder. Mix gently to coat the tofu evenly and avoid breaking up the tofu cubes.
3. Heat oil in a frying pan or wok over medium-high heat. Add the coated tofu and fry, stirring often, until the cubes are evenly golden-brown and crispy on all sides.

Set aside.

Garlicky Cashew Broccoli:

1. Stir together brown sugar and hot water until sugar is dissolved. Add soy sauce and lemon juice. Set aside.
2. In the same frying pan or wok used to cook the tofu, heat 1 ½ tbsp. vegan butter over high heat. Add the broccoli florets and stir-fry uncovered, for 2-3 minutes. Cover and cook for another 2-3 minutes, until the florets are nearly tender.
3. Add another ½ tbsp. vegan butter, cashews, and minced garlic. Stir well and cook for another 1-2 minutes (until garlic is cooked and fragrant.)

4. Add the tofu and the brown sugar/soy sauce mixture. Mix well and cook for another 1-2 minutes, until the sauce reduced.
5. Serve over couscous. Add sesame seeds and sriracha to taste.

Prep Time: 20 Minutes

Cook Time: 35 Minutes

Servings: 2

Ingredient

Spicy Potatoes & Chickpeas:

- 2 cups The Little Potato Company's Little Reds, quartered
- 1 cup canned chickpeas, drained
- 2 tsp olive oil
- 1 tbsp sriracha
- ½ tsp garlic powder
- ½ tsp onion powder
- ½ tsp turmeric
- ¼ tsp salt

Roasted Carrots:

- 1 cup carrots, sliced diagonally
- 1 tsp olive oil
- 1 tsp maple syrup
- ¼ tsp garlic powder
- ½ tsp turmeric
- ¼ tsp paprika
- pinch salt

Zucchini:

- 1 zucchini, sliced
- 1 tsp olive oil

- pinch of salt and pepper

Garlicky Sautéed Kale:

- 1 bunch kale, destemmed and roughly chopped
- 2 tsp olive oil
- 1 clove garlic, minced
- 1 tsp lemon juice
- pinch of salt and pepper

Hummus Dressing:

- 1 tbsp hummus
- 1 tbsp tahini
- 2 tbsp water
- 2 tsp lemon juice
- ½ tsp garlic powder
- 1 tbsp nutritional yeast
- 1 tsp olive oil
- pinch salt

Instructions

Roasted Vegetables:

1. Spicy Potatoes & Chickpeas: Preheat oven to 425F. Combine all ingredients in a medium bowl and mix well. Transfer to a sheet pan lined with parchment paper.
2. Roasted Carrots: In the same bowl used above, combine the carrots, olive oil, garlic powder, turmeric, paprika, maple syrup, and salt. Mix well and transfer to the sheet pan from the previous step.

3. Zucchini: Using the same bowl, combine the zucchini, olive oil, and a sprinkle of salt and pepper, mix well. Transfer to the sheet pan.
4. Roasting: Bake everything for 15 minutes. Flip/stir everything and bake for another 15-20 minutes, until potatoes are tender and chickpeas are crisp.

Garlicky Sautéed Kale:

1. Preheat olive oil in a large skillet over medium-high heat. Add the minced garlic and kale. Sauté, stirring often, until kale wilts. Sprinkle kale with 1 teaspoon lemon juice, and a pinch of salt and pepper. Continue sautéing until kale is tender. Taste and adjust seasoning if necessary.

Hummus Dressing

2. Combine all ingredients (in a blender or using a whisk.) Thin with water if necessary. Taste and adjust seasoning.

Serving:

3. Divide kale between 2 bowls. Top each bowl with ½ of the roasted potatoes, ½ of the carrots, and ½ of the zucchini. Top with ½ of the chickpeas and a drizzle of hummus dressing.

Prep Time: 20 Minutes

Cook Time: 1hr 40 Minutes

Servings: 1

Ingredient

Pumpkin Pie Filling:

- 1 ½ cups pure pumpkin puree
- 1 cup evaporated cane sugar
- ¼ tsp salt
- ¼ tsp vanilla extract
- ¼ tsp pumpkin pie spice
- ½ tsp cinnamon
- ⅔ cup almond or soy milk
- 2 tbsp coconut cream
- 2 tbsp ground flax seed
- 3 tbsp cornstarch

Oat Crisp Pie Crust:

- 1 cup + 2 tbsp oats
- ⅔ cup whole wheat flour
- ⅓ cup brown sugar
- ⅓ cup vegan butter
- 2 tbsp water
- 2 tbsp ground flax seed
- ¼ tsp cinnamon
- ⅛ Tsp salt

Coconut Whip:

- 1 can high-quality canned coconut cream
- ¼ tsp vanilla
- 1 tbsp maple syrup

Instructions

Pie Filling + Oat Crisp Crust:

4. Preheat your oven to 300F.
5. In a medium-large bowl whisk together all of the filling ingredients. Refrigerate for 15 minutes while you work on the crust.
6. Combine all of the crust ingredients. Use your hands or a pastry blender to break up the vegan butter into pea-sized or smaller pieces. Squeeze a little bit of dough in your hand to see if it holds together. Add a few teaspoons of water if it's too dry.
7. Drop about ¾ of the dough into your pie plate (I used a 10" non-stick tart pan.) Use your fingers to evenly press the dough flat. Use the remaining ¼ of the dough to build the crust up the sides by about ¾". Try to avoid making the corners too thick.
8. Bake the crust at 300F for 10 minutes.
9. After the crust has baked, pour the filling into the crust and use a spatula to even out the surface. Bake for 1 hour and 40 minutes, or until the small cracks form around the outer edges of the fillings and the center is dry to the touch.
10. Let the pie cool at room temperature before chilling in the refrigerator.
11. Serve with coconut whipped cream!

Coconut Whipped Cream:

1. Simply place your canned coconut cream in the fridge until well chilled. Then, turn the can upside down and open the "bottom" of the can. With good quality coconut cream, half of the can should be a thick coconut milk and the other half should be a thick, dense layer of coconut cream.
2. Scoop the thick cream into a bowl, add a dash of vanilla extract and 2 tablespoon maple syrup.
3. Whip on high until light and fluffy.

Prep Time: 1hr 3 Minutes

Cook Time: 40 Minutes

Servings: 6

Ingredient

- 1 tbsp (15 ml) olive oil
- 1 ½ cups kale, shredded and tightly packed
- 1 medium-large carrot, grated
- ½ onion, finely chopped
- 1 rib celery, thinly sliced
- 3 cloves garlic, minced
- 1 ½ cups mushrooms, thinly sliced
- 1 tsp (5 ml) salt, to taste
- ¼ tsp (1.25 ml) oregano
- ¼ tsp (1.25 ml) thyme

Black pepper, to taste:

- 1 cup overcooked green lentils
- 1 cup cooked brown rice
- ½ cup ground walnuts
- ⅓ cup oat flour (ground oats)
- 3 tbsp ground flax seed
- 2 tablespoons nutritional yeast
- ¼ cup dried cranberries (optional)
- ½ cup (125 ml) cranberry sauce, canned or homemade (recipe below)

Instructions

1. Preheat your oven to 400°F (200°C).
2. In a large frying pan heat olive oil over medium-high. Once the oil is hot, add the kale, carrot, onion, celery, and garlic. Sauté until the onion is nearly translucent (about 2 minutes).
3. Add the mushrooms, salt, oregano, thyme, and pepper. Sauté until the vegetables are just tender.
4. In a large bowl, combine the vegetables, cooked lentils and brown rice, walnuts, oat flour, flax seed, and nutritional yeast. Mix thoroughly and roughly, mashing some of the ingredients in the process. This is important to help the loaf bind together.
5. If needed, blend ⅓ of the mixture using a food processor or immersion blender and recombine. For best texture and appearance do not blend all of the mixture.
6. If using, mix in the dried cranberries. Taste and adjust seasoning with salt and pepper.
7. Line a loaf pan with parchment paper and firmly press the mixture into the pan.
8. Bake for 25 minutes. While the loaf bakes, prepare the cranberry glaze: In a high-speed blender, blend the cranberry sauce until smooth. Remove the loaf from the oven, pour the glaze over the top and bake for an additional 10-15 minutes, until the glaze has set and no longer looks shiny.
9. Allow the loaf to cool for 10-15 minutes to fully set.
10. Store leftovers for up to 4 days.

Prep Time: 20 Minutes

Cook Time: 15 Minutes

Servings: 24

Ingredient

- Ivies or green onions
- sriracha
- vegan mayo or sour cream
- fresh dill
- black pepper

Instructions

1. Preheat oven to 400F.
2. Prick each potato with a fork 2-3 times. (Don't worry about washing these guys,it's already been done for you!)
3. Microwave on HIGH for 5 minutes.
4. Toss the hot potatoes in olive oil, garlic powder, salt, and pepper. Bake for 8 minutes before flipping and then bake for an addition 5- 10 minutes. Poke them with a knife to check if they're tender.
5. Once they're cooked, let them sit for 5-10 minutes until they're just cool enough to handle. Deeply score each potato both lengthwise and width wise.
6. Using your index fingers and thumbs, gently pinch and push the corners of each potato inwards to mash and fluff the cooked centers out of the potato. (Refer to the 4th set of pictures for a visual reference)

7. Drop a part of vegan butter into the center of each potato followed by a big pinch of vegan cheese.
8. Place under the broiler just long enough for the cheese to melt and bubble.

Toppings:

1. For Tex-Mex potatoes: Top with a dollop of guacamole, a little drizzle of sriracha or taco sauce, and a sprinkle of chives or green onions.
2. For "Loaded Baked Potatoes": Top with a teeny dollop of vegan mayo or sour cream, a sprinkle of dill and chives, and black pepper.

Prep Time: 20 Minutes

Cook Time: 1hr 20 Minutes

Servings: 5

Ingredient

- 1 Tofurky Roast, thawed in fridge for 24 hours

For The Baste:

- 3 tablespoons (45 ml) olive oil
- 2 tablespoons (30 ml) soy sauce
- 1 tablespoon (15 ml) maple syrup
- 1 clove garlic, minced
- 1.5 teaspoons each of fresh chopped thyme, oregano, sage, and rosemary (for dried herbs, use ½ teaspoon each or sub with 2 teaspoons dried poultry or Italian seasoning - rubbed not ground)

Vegetables (Optional)

- 1 medium sweet potato, peeled and chopped
- 1-2 carrots, peeled and chopped
- 6-10 Creamer potatoes, halved

For The Gravy (Optional)

- Tofurky "drippings"
- 3 tablespoons (35 grams) flour
- 2 cups (500 ml) vegetable broth

Instructions

Tofurky Roast and Vegetables:

1. Preheat your oven to 350°F (180°C).
2. Use a knife or scissors to carefully cut off one of the end clips. Run the thawed Tofurky Roast under warm water as you loosen and remove the plastic.
3. Prepare the baste in a small bowl. Mix together olive oil, soy sauce, maple syrup, minced garlic, and herbs.
4. If cooking vegetables, toss them with 3 tablespoons of baste. Arrange vegetables in your baking dish.
5. Put a piece of parchment paper in the center of your baking dish. Add the Tofurky Roast and cover with half of the baste.
6. Note: If cooking vegetables in the same dish as the Tofurky, the parchment paper barrier prevents the vegetables from simmering in the excess baste, overcooking and over-seasoning them. The parchment makes it easier to reserve the Tofurky "drippings" for making vegan gravy.
7. Cover the baking dish tightly with aluminum foil.
8. Cook for 1 hour and 20 minutes. Check for doneness at 1 hour. Once the vegetables are nearly tender and the Tofurky is golden-brown, pour the remaining baste over the Tofurky and cook, uncovered, for an additional 10-15 minutes. Cook until the vegetables are tender and the Tofurky Roast reaches an internal temperature of 165°F (75°C).
9. Optional: Reserve excess baste or Tofurky "drippings" for making vegan gravy.
10. Use a very sharp or serrated knife to thinly slice the Tofurky Roast for serving.

Tofurky Gravy:

1. Heat the Tofurky "drippings" in a small saucepan over medium heat. Once hot, make a roux by whisking in 3 tablespoons of flour. Add a splash of the vegetable broth if the roux is too thick to stir. Cook, stirring constantly for 1-2 minutes. Whisk in the vegetable broth, slowly and gradually, to prevent lumps.
2. Simmer until your desired consistency is reached (the gravy will thicken slightly as it cools.)
3. Taste and adjust the consistency and seasoning using vegetable broth, water, salt, and pepper.

Prep Time: 15 Minutes

Cook Time: 10 Minutes

Servings: 4

Ingredient

Lentil + Chickpea Salad:

- 1 cup cooked red lentils
- 1 cup chickpeas, canned (drained)
- 1 celery rib, finely chopped
- 1 carrot, grated
- ¼ red or green bell pepper, finely chopped (optional)
- 2-3 green onions, finely chopped
- 1 medium pickle, finely chopped
- 3 tbsp fresh dill, finely chopped
- ½ tbsp lemon juice
- 3-4 tablespoon vegan mayo (I use 4) (or sub for hummus)
- 2-3 tablespoon nutritional yeast (I use 3)
- ¼ tsp black salt
- black pepper, to taste

Lentil + Chickpea Salad Sandwich

- 2 slices of sprouted, whole grain, or gluten free bread
- ⅓-½ cup of lentil + chickpea salad
- 1-2 leaves of lettuce (butter, romaine, spinach, or iceberg)

Instructions

1. Wash, chop and prepare all ingredients. Make sure the vegetables are chopped nice and fine. Feel free to use the chop/slice function on your food processor.
2. Lightly mash chickpeas with a fork. Add the lentils, finely chopped vegetables, mayo, lemon juice, nutritional yeast, black salt, and pepper. Mix thoroughly with a fork.
3. Blend ⅓-1/2 of the mixture with an immersion blender (or use the pulse function on your food processor). Mix thoroughly with a fork to even out the texture.
4. Optional: Chill for 3+ hours before serving.

Lentil + Chickpea Salad Sandwich:

1. Scoop ⅓-1/2 cup of Lentil + Chickpea Salad on one slice of bread and lay 2 leaves of lettuce on the other slice of bread. Close the sandwich, slice diagonally and enjoy!

Prep Time: 30 Minutes

Cook Time: 10 Minutes

Servings: 2

Ingredient

Grilled Veggies:

- ⅔ cup zucchini, halved and sliced
- ⅔ cup sliced bell peppers (red, green and yellow)
- ¼ red onion, thin sliced
- ⅔ cup sliced mushrooms
- 1 handful baby spinach, roughly chopped
- ¼ tsp salt

Taco Rice & Beans:

- 1 ⅓ cups cooked white or brown rice
- ⅔ cup black beans, rinsed and drained
- 3 tbsp taco sauce

Toppings:

- 1 vine-ripened tomato, chopped
- 1 handful baby spinach, roughly chopped
- 2-4 tablespoon guacamole
- 2-4 tablespoon salsa
- 2+ handfuls of tortilla chips

Toppings More Optional:

- ¼ cup Daiya Mozzarella, Cheddar, or Pepper jack style shreds

- Fresh lime juice or wedges
- Extra taco sauce for drizzling
- Jalapeño, thin sliced
- Cilantro, chopped
- Salsa baked tofu

Instructions

2. Bine cooked rice, rinsed black beans, and taco sauce in a microwave-safe container. Heat on high for 3-4 minutes or until hot.
3. Preheat grill or skillet (high heat). Spray with non-stick cooking spray or brush with vegetComable oil (about 2-3 tsp.)
4. Cook bell pepper, red onion, and zucchini for about 4 min. Add mushrooms, sprinkle with salt and cook for another 5-6 minutes or until veggies are tender. Add spinach and cook until just wilted.
5. To serve: Scoop ¾ cup of rice and bean mixture into a bowl and add ½ of the grilled veggies. Top with a handful of fresh greens (iceberg lettuce or spinach), fresh chopped tomato, 2+ handfuls of crushed tortilla chips, 1-2 tablespoon of guacamole, and 1-2 tablespoon of salsa. Add any optional topping you desire (fresh cilantro, Daiya cheese, fresh lime juice, salsa baked tofu, extra taco sauce, etc.)

Prep Time: 20 Minutes

Cook Time: 45 Minutes

Servings: 6

Ingredient

Marinade & Glaze:

- ¼ cup maple syrup
- 3 tbsp soy sauce
- 2 tbsp bbq sauce
- 1 tbsp sriracha
- ½ tbsp olive oil
- Pinch garlic powder

Veggie Skewers:

- ½ package The Little Potato Company's Oven | BBQ Ready Kits in Garlic or BBQ Blend
- 1 454g package of extra-firm pressed tofu
- 1 small zucchini chopped into large chunks
- 1 large bell pepper cut into large chunks (I used a mix of red, green and yellow for extra color)
- 4-5 large mushrooms cut into extra-large chunks (leave small mushrooms whole)
- ¼ red onion cut into large chunks

Instructions

1. Mix together marinade ingredients. Chop tofu into large ¾" -1" cubes. Marinate the tofu for 1-2 hours. After marinating, preheat your oven to 450F.
2. Prepare your choice of The Little Potato Company's Oven | BBQ Ready Kits according to the package instructions. Place the foil tray on a large baking tray. Bake for 10 minutes.
3. After 10 minutes, move the tray of potatoes to one side of the baking tray. Line the other side of the baking tray with parchment paper and arrange the marinated tofu cubes. Reserve any excess marinade. Bake for 15 minutes. Flip the tofu and stir the potatoes before baking for another 10 minutes.
4. While the tofu and potatoes bake, heat the remaining marinade in a small saucepan over medium heat. Simmer gently for 5 minutes or until slightly thickened.
5. Spray or brush preheated grill with a light coat of oil. Lightly precook the vegetables for about 5 minutes until just barely tender. Season with a light sprinkle of salt during cooking.
6. Beginning and ending with a piece of tofu or potato (this will prevent veggies from slipping off the skewers), alternate skewering a variety of veggies, tofu, and potatoes, making sure to have an equal amount of each food per skewer.
7. Brush assembled skewers with glaze and grill until veggies are tender. Pour any remaining glaze over skewers and serve.

Prep Time: 5 Minutes

Cook Time: 5 Minutes

Servings: 2

Ingredient

The Best Green Smoothie:

- 1 cup unsweetened almond or soy milk
- 1-2 handfuls of spinach
- 2 frozen bananas
- 2-4 soft pitted dates
- 2 tbsp hemp hearts
- 1 tbsp natural peanut butter
- 2 ice cubes

Super food Smoothie Topping (Optional)

- 2 tbsp hemp seeds
- 2 tbsp chia seeds
- 2 tbsp raw buckwheat grouts
- 2 tbsp slivered almonds (or pumpkin seeds)

Instructions

The Best Green Smoothie:

1. Combine all ingredients, blend on high until perfectly smooth and frothy.

Super food Smoothie Topping (Optional)

2. Combine all ingredients. Sprinkle 1 tablespoon on top of your smoothie.

73

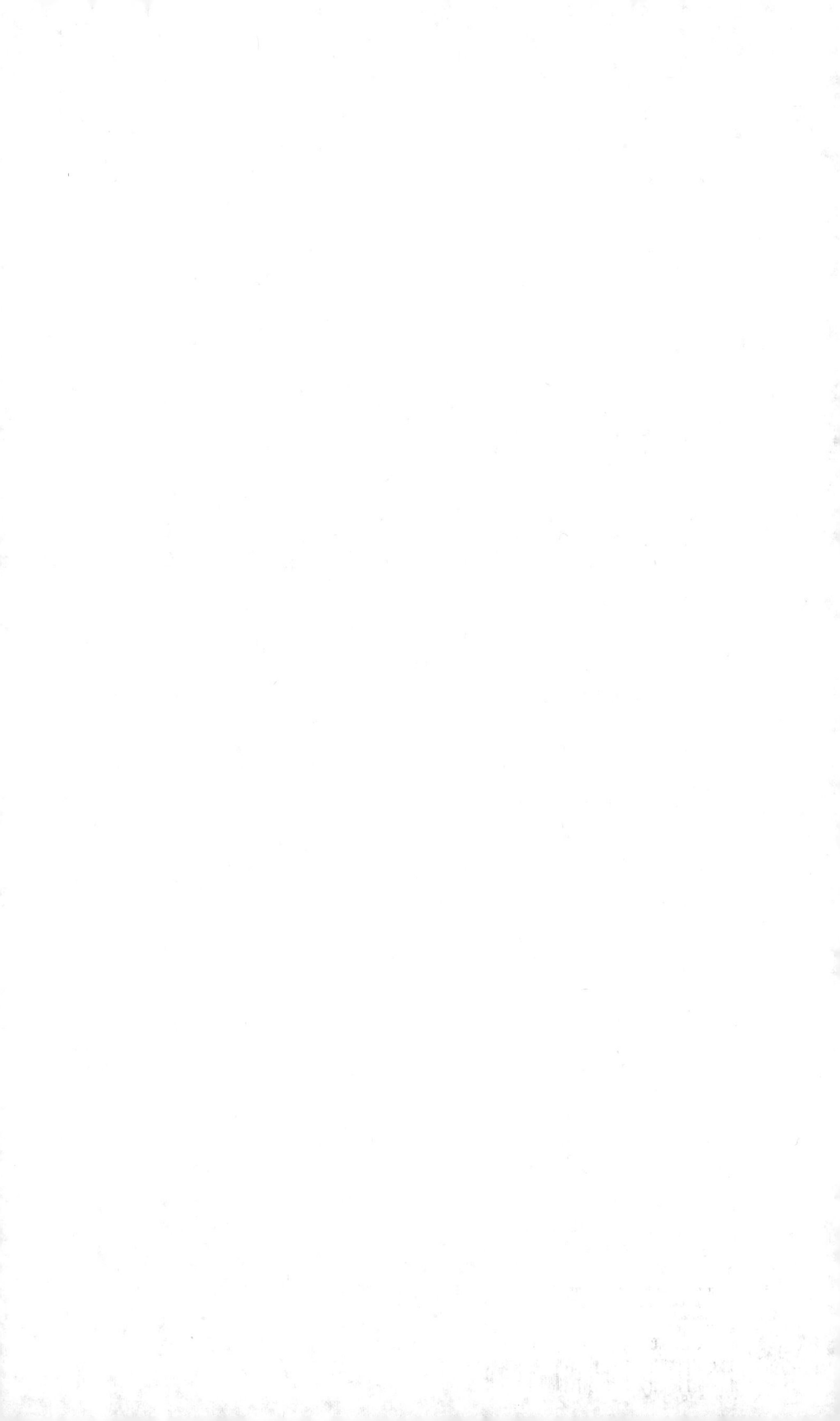